Meatless Recipes and Healthy Food Choices

By Doris Richardson-Edsell

Copyright by Doris Richardson- Edsell, April 2014

Dedicated to people who want to move toward healthier eating through a plant based diet

Table of Contents

About the Author

Doris Richardson-Edsell is a registered nurse, yoga teacher, mother and grandmother who has authored over 15 books on Amazon.com. She writes daily on her website: Body Mind Health. www.body-mindhealth.com. Doris is a strong advocate for people with emotional difficulties.

Dedicated to those who seek healthy living in mind, body and soul.

What is your best food group?

Fruits and veggies are the best food group for you to stay healthy and well

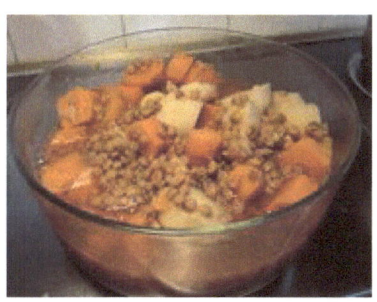

Lentil soup with sweet and white potatoes is a good healthy choice. The lentils are packed with protein and the sweet potatoes full of vitamins and minerals

Fruits and vegetables are packed with fiber and vitamins for your health. If you are trying to get healthier or lose some weight, add more fruits and veggies to your daily diet.

What is Nutrition?

The term- Nutrition means to nourish and good nutrition promotes health and well-being in mind, body and spirit. Good nutritious foods provide energy to the body and foods are divided into carbohydrates, fats and proteins. There are 2 kinds of carbohydrates; the simple sugars (which you should have in limited portions) and the complex carbs– our starches from our grains such as rice, quinoa, barley and oats, potatoes, and don't forget that yellow corn is a grain too. Carbohydrates are also our fruits and vegetables. Carbohydrates provide the fuel you need to heat your body and the energy we need to start our day. That is why oatmeal would be a great choice for your morning energy.

You do need some dietary fat in daily foods but not as much as you may be eating. And remember to stay away from the dietary fat that is saturated fat (from butter, lard, processed foods- even candy!) and stick to the unsaturated fat because the good fats contain the essential fatty acids that we need for health and wellness. Adding just a teaspoon of olive oil to your diet each day can help. There really is no need for adding supplements such as fish oil to your diet unless you do not get enough essential fatty acids from the foods you eat.

Proteins- You may know that protein is for tissue building and it is a necessary component of a healthy diet. These amino acids are the building blocks of for making and repairing body tissues. There are ways to get your protein without always eating meat. Learn how to cook tofu and tempeh, great sources of protein along with grains; most grains have 9 grams of protein per 1/4 cup serving, and black eyed peas and all the beans and legumes (such as split peas and lentils) are packed with protein too.

Vitamins and Minerals

And for tissue repair do not forget about minerals and vitamins. Vitamins are essential to certain tissues. For example, Vitamin C helps to produce the substance that cements tissues together to prevent tissue bleeding and Vitamin A is in the rods and cones of your eyes for vision in dim light.

As for the minerals, we need minerals to give strength to our bones and teeth- this is found in calcium. And the trace element iron is a component of hemoglobin to bind oxygen for cell transport.

Reference from topics of Nutrition: Schlenker &Roth (2011) *Williams Essentials of Nutrition and Diet Therapy*. Tenth Ed. St. Louis, Mo., Elsevier-Mosby

[Parsnips and Potatoes](#)

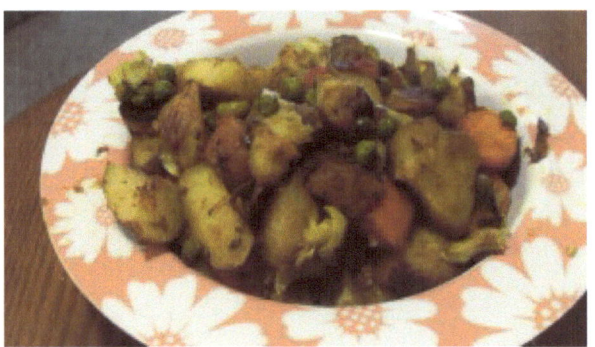

Trying something new is a great thing- this week add parsnips to your veggies mix!

I recently started using parsnips in my recipes because I tried them and really enjoy eating them. They look like carrots except parsnips are white.

An easy recipe that I made in a frying pan and I just peeled and chopped 2 carrots, 2 parsnips and 1 potato (left -over cooked the day before). I also chopped a tomato and a slice of pineapple, and added a cup of frozen peas.

In a frying pan I added a teaspoon of olive oil and teaspoon of fresh chopped ginger and then added the carrots, the chopped tomato and parsnips for about 10 minutes. (The tomato adds the moisture for the steaming effect).

Use your own judgment on how you like your carrots and parsnips- I like mine crisp so I cook for about 8 minutes.

Afterwards I added the peas and the pineapple and already cooked cubed potato; cooking for another 5 minutes.

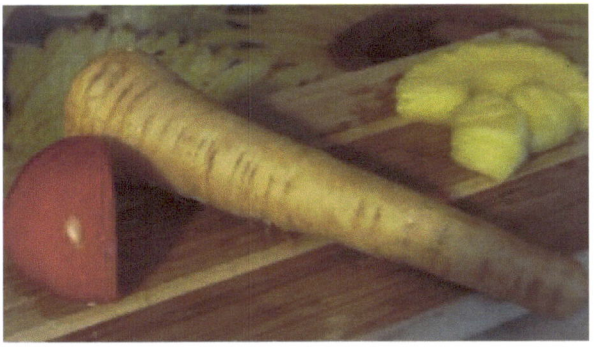

Parsnips-the other carrot!

While cooking for some added zest, I added a sprinkle of Cumin and Turmeric for some added color and flavor. This is growing evidence on spices adding to your health and Turmeric was just reviewed for help in Alzheimer Disease- helping with memory.

Loving What Your Eat, and Eating What You Love

Organization is the key to a great healthy living plan

Have a clean kitchen where it is a pleasure to make meals; your counters are clean, and you have enough food in you fridge to create great, low calorie meals with plenty of fruits and vegetables.

More of the good Carbs Please!

What are the good carbs? They are the ones that take a long time to get through your body; rice, grains, fruits and vegetables. They are the color in your meals; the bright red bell peppers, the fresh orange carrots and the greener than green collard greens! You can eat them raw, you can eat them blanched, and you can eat them in soups. And veggies should be your main staple because you can eat as much as you want!

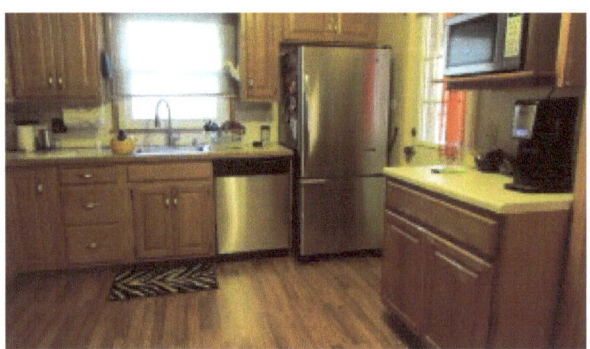

Organize your kitchen so that everything is where it needs to be. Make it a clean environment where you can make a nice meal

When I think of eating, I think of fresh fruits and veggies. I love to eat a variety of foods that are colorful and tasty. Crispy veggies with some brown rice are a great meal. If you begin to enjoy the low fat- complex carbohydrates instead of the fatty foods, you really begin to enjoy what you are eating.

Taking control
Begin to take control of your eating by only eating when you are hungry. Many people go by the clock with eating. Allow your body to tell you when it needs care.

Activity
When you are active every day of your life, you learn the cues of your body's hunger. You become hungry because you are moving and grooving!

Realism
If you are trying to lose some weight, stop punishing yourself with unrealistic goals of losing a lot of weight. Make mini goals of losing 3 pounds, not 20. The pounds will come off if you stick to it.

Your body size

You need to begin cherishing the way you look even if you are not where you want to be. Striving for perfection is not the key to long lasting weight control. And looking at the commercials on TV telling you that you can be a 10 may be very unrealistic. Do not send yourself critical messages about your body; love your body.

Be Mindful

Always be mindful of eating. Do not sit in front of the TV eating because this one thing will sabotage all your efforts for your day.

Eat slowly and mindfully, small bits of food cut up, whatever you need to do to slow you down. Look at your food, use colorful, small plates that exaggerate how much you are eating, and of course- chew your food well.

What are you eating? Some Functional Foods

There are many foods which are packed with vitamins and minerals to help you stay healthy and well. Did you know that they are called Functional Foods?

The first Functional Food that I think about are the orange ones! Carotenoids- they are the B-Carotene in carrots, orange fruits, butternut squash and cantaloupe. Great for your health and wellness; the yellower the better!

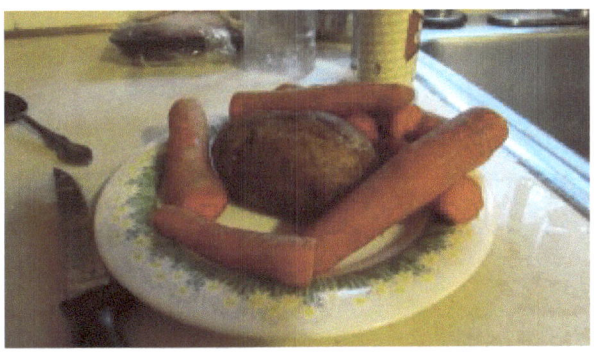

Back to basics; steamed carrots and potatoes

Here are a few more functional foods:

Lycopene is found in foods such as tomato products.

Lutein is found in dark green veggies such as kale, spinach, collard greens, eggs, corn and citrus.

Onions, garlic, scallions, leeks and chives are called-
Diallyl Sulfides and the name for strawberries,
raspberries, pomegranates, and berries and walnuts are
called- Ellagic Acids

OMEGA 3's

And you have all heard of the Omega – 3 s and how
important they are. You do not have to take these fatty
acids in pill form if you eat them. The fatty acid- a-
linolenic acid is found in flax seeds, flax oil, walnuts,
canola oil, soybean oil, sardines in oil and Atlantic
salmon.

For some Eicosapentaenoic Acid- you can eat some
herring, salmon, Wild Alaskan Salmon, blue fin tuna.

And finally, you can find Docosahexaenoic Acid in
Atlantic salmon, Blue Fin Tuna, Mackerel and Omega-3
enriched eggs.

And if it sounds complicated, it really is not. Here are
some tips on how to get your pre and probiotics.

PREBIOTIC- Whole grains, especially oatmeal, flax
and barley, greens, berries, bananas, legumes, onions,
garlic, honey and leeks.

PROBIOTIC- This is your yogurt. But it does not have
to be only dairy yogurt. You can find probiotics in soy,
almond or coconut yogurt, and fermented dairy and non-
dairy products such as sauerkraut and fermented soy such
as meso and tempeh.

Other functional Foods:

Phenols- they are in apples, pears, citrus fruit, parsley, carrots, broccoli, cabbage, cucumbers, squash, yams and tomatoes.

Lignans- they are found in flax seed, rye

Flavonoids- found in berries, especially the dark berries, cherries, red grapes and tea– especially green tea.

Your diet and what you should be eating

When you are choosing what to eat, you want to stick to the basics such as discovering the resources that are available to you such as Getting Started with *My Plate*. It replaced the food pyramid a few years ago, making it easier to understand what you should be eating. This government program is online for your convenience-
ChooseMyPlate.gov

The recommendations on healthy eating include:

Enjoy your food but eat less

Avoid oversized portions

Make half of your plate fruits and veggies!

Switch to fat free or low fat milk (1%)

Make at least half of your grains– whole grains

Look at the sodium in foods- especially products such as soups, breads and frozen meals, and choose foods with low sodium numbers

Drink water instead of sugary drinks

Taken from the US government resource: MyPlate.gov. Fall/Winter 2011

What to do with Kale? Mix With Beans and Grains

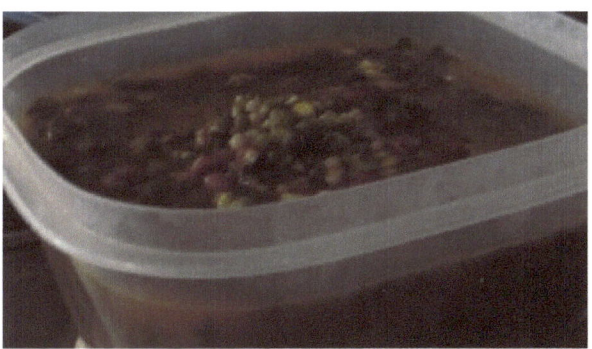

The beauty of making soup is that it can help you with increasing the fiber in your diet.

Did you know that there are many studies on the fact that people who eat soup are thinner?

Veggie Soup with Split peas and beans

Some recipes that are good and packed with protein include adding grains, legumes and beans.
Here is a recipe for a great veggie soup with kidney beans, split peas and kale.

For many people who are sodium restricted, making your own soup is a very good idea because you alone control the amount of salt you put in. And there are many different kinds of spices that you can use in a recipe that perk up the flavor without adding any salt.

For most of my soup recipes, I start out in a separate frying pan sprinkled with 2 teaspoons of olive oil, adding teaspoon of very finely chopped ginger, a clove of chopped garlic, and 1 small chopped white onion. I simmer for about 5 minutes and put to the side to add to my soup.

Starting the Soup

I always start out with 2 cups of tomato or V-8 juice, adding 2 cups of water or veggie broth. Remember to use the low sodium kind, especially if you are on a sodium restricted diet.

I add the onion, garlic and ginger and then I begin to add 1/2 cup raw soy beans, 1/2 cup quinoa, 1/2 cup split peas (they need to be rinsed thoroughly for stones/bugs) first because they take about 1/2 hour to cook. After the grains, legumes and soy beans are almost done, I begin to add my other veggies such as 2 cups fresh kale, 1 cup frozen corn, 1 can of kidney beans, rinsed well.

Simmer for another 30 minutes or longer depending on how you like your veggies.

Each cup of this soup is packed with fiber and protein.

Kale Chips

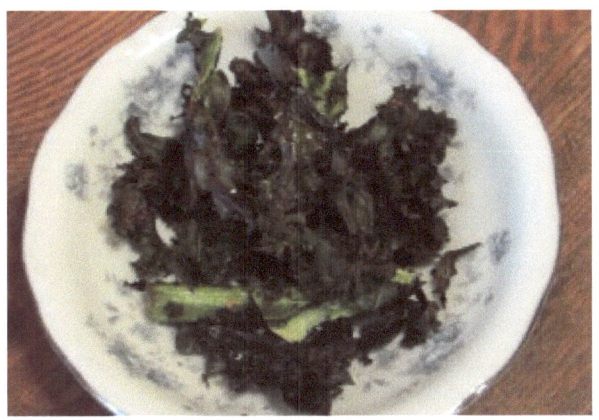

Crunchy like potato chips!

For an added appetizer, I also roast some kale in the oven.

Use some Canola cooking spray on a cookie sheet. Add washed and dry pieces of kale to the cookie sheet, sprinkle with garlic powder and a little salt and cook in an over 350 degrees for about 10 minutes. Let set for about 5 minutes and eat as a snack or as an appetizer for your soup.

Do you want healthy digestion? Focus on good food combinations

A Healthy diet and exercise can deliver you great health

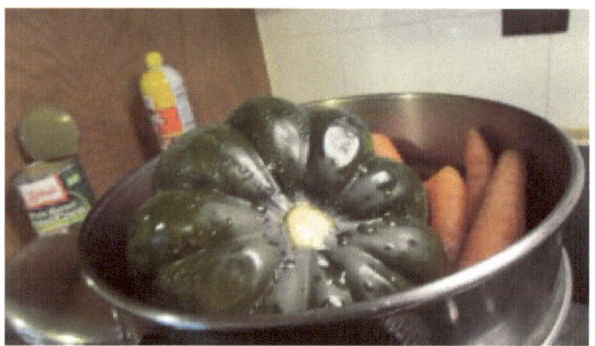

Some steamed veggies, great for your health and wellness

Today there are many new diet and exercise tips but good nutrition tips have been around for many years.
Author Dr. Howard Hay developed The Hay Diet in 1939 and his theories are still very sound advice today.

The theory is on the importance of food combinations for healthy digestion.

Dr. Hay pointed out that a combination of high-protein and high-starch foods has appalling effects on the digestive system. Dr. Hay himself was troubled by painful digestion for many years related to chronic inflammation of his kidneys, high blood pressure and a badly dilated heart. When he changed his eating habits, his symptoms disappeared.23

Here is Dr. Hay's General Theory on Food: The Hay Diet

1. Carbohydrates should never be eaten in combination with proteins and acidic foods

2. Vegetables, salads and fruits should make up the bulk of the diet

3. Proteins, carbohydrates and fats should be eaten only in small amounts. Only wholegrain, unrefined carbohydrates should be used

4. Refined and processed foods should be avoided

5. There should be an interval of at least 4 hours between meals of different types of foods

6. One meal a day should be based on starchy foods, another on protein foods and the third should be alkaline foods. Some alkaline foods have a neutral pH such as tap water, most spring water. A pH of 8 foods- apples almonds, grapefruit, corn, mushrooms, turnip, soy, bell pepper, radish, pineapple, cherries, wild rice, apricot, strawberries, bananas. pH 9- avocado, green tea, lettuce, celery, peas, sweet potatoes, eggplant, green beans, beets, blueberries, pears, grapes, Kiwi, tangerines, figs, dates, mangoes, papaya pH 10- spinach, broccoli, artichoke, Brussels sprouts, cabbage, cauliflower, carrots,

cucumber, lemon, limes, seaweed, asparagus, radish, collard greens, onions.

ACIDIC FOODS THAT CAUSE DIGESTIVE ISSUES– carbonated water, club soda, energy drinks– pH3

pH 4 Popcorn, cream cheese, buttermilk, prunes, pastries, cheese, pork, beer, wine, black tea, pickles, chocolate, roasted nuts, vinegar, sweet and low, equal, nutra sweet.

pH 5 Purified water, distilled water, coffee, sweetened fruit juice, pistachios, beef, white bread, peanuts, nuts, wheat

pH 6- Most grains, eggs, fish, tea, cooked beans, cooked spinach, soy milk, coconut, lima beans, plums, brown rice, barley, cocoa, oats, liver, oyster, salmon.

What is really causing your indigestion or bloating?

Indigestion is caused by too much acid in the stomach. What to avoid: Alcohol, strong tea, coffee, fizzy drinks. meat extracts, acidic foods such as pickles and vinegar, hot spicy foods, unripe fruit, cheese.

Discomfort or bloating?

Other common triggers of digestive issues are stress, eating too fast or hurried, insufficient chewing, long gaps between meals which leads to binge eating; swallowing air, and bloating. Tobacco use also triggers gastric acid secretion.

The basic principles of the Hay Diet:

1. Understand that starch begins to ferment in the stomach as soon as the salivary enzyme ptyalin is destroyed by gastric juices

2. Healthy foods in the right combinations can greatly improve digestion

3. All foods comprise of one of the 5 nutrients and it is vital to identify the dominant nutrient in a meal, and proportion accordingly:

THE 5 NUTRIENT GROUPS

Starches- bread, pasta rice

Proteins- meat, fish, eggs cheese, soy

Sugars- firm fruit such as fresh banana, honey, sweet preserves

Acids- soft fruits such as peaches, plums

Fats- oil, mayonnaise, egg yolk

Carbohydrates fall into 2 groups- the sugars and starches.

Example: Remember that proteins, carbs and fats should be eaten in small amounts. Veggies, salads and fruits make up the bulk of your diet with 4 hours between meals.

Breakfast (starch)

Oatmeal with almond milk (carbs)

Sliced banana and pineapple

Lunch (based on protein)

Soy burger (9 grams protein), slice wholegrain bread, lettuce salad with raw veggies such as cucumbers, celery and carrots.

Dinner (alkaline food focused)

Veggie mix of broccoli, red bell peppers, and 1/2 cup brown rice (limited portion of rice- a healthy carb). Fruit cup of mangoes and papaya are a bit acidic due to their soft nature.

Snack- apple- hard fruit the best for low acidity

Exercise

Do not forget about exercise in your healthy living plan. Exercise such as a fast walk in the morning helps the digestion of foods in the body.

Tips on some food combos and indigestion from the book by: Dries, J. & Dries, I (2002) *The Food Combining Bible.* Hammersmith, London. Harper-Collins.

What is in your refrigerator?

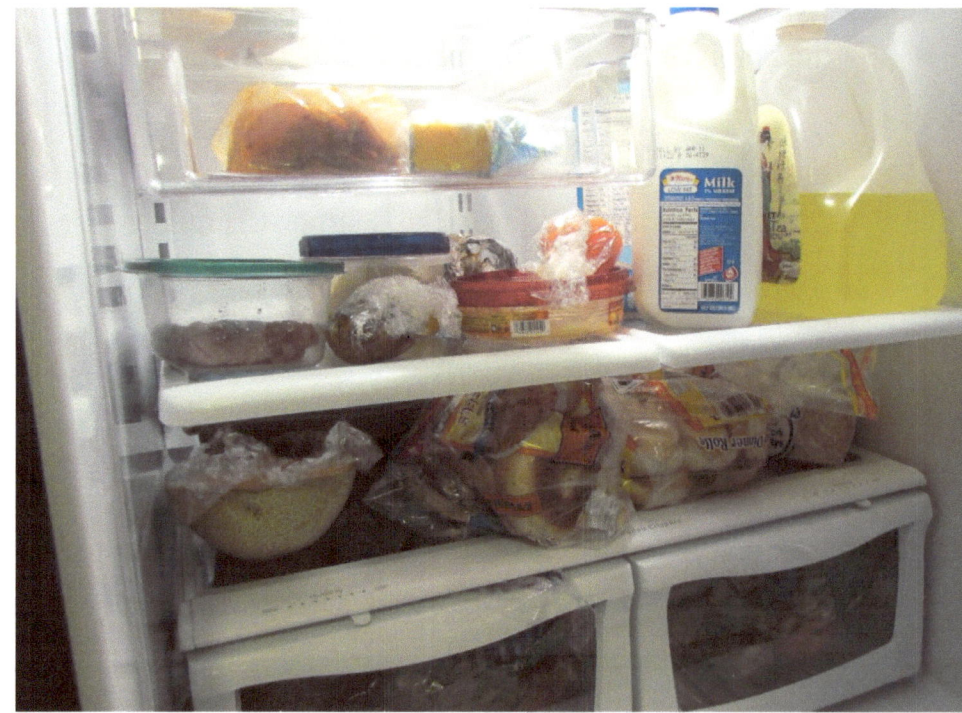

What is in your refrigerator is a good question for you to ponder

 Take a look at this refrigerator. There are some good and bad things here. The first thing that I see is the ketchup. Condiments such as ketchup have high fructose corn syrup which is very bad for you. All condiments have their disadvantages; tasting good but too much sodium, fat or sugar. (Mustard=sodium and mayonnaise=fat). There is low fat mayonnaise and low sodium mustards but you have to begin reading labels. I believe that there may be ketchup on the market without high fructose corn syrup.

I also see some white bread; this should also be replaced with whole grain bread. In the top tray is cheese and pepperoni; another sabotage to a healthy diet.

Good things: ½ cantaloupe, low fat milk, hummus, ½ tomato, lettuce in the bottom tray along with some carrots. There are also apples, a grapefruit and some oranges in the bottom tray on the right.

The juice in the refrigerator that looks yellow is coconut-pineapple Dansani water enhancer; a better choice that soda.

Decide for yourself what is important to you in your healthy living plan. You may need to indulge in some extras that you see here, but not all the time if you want to stay healthy in mind, body and spirit.

Simple side dishes packed with vitamins- The Acorn Squash

Do you want something simple, low calorie and easy to make? Try some acorn squash. You can steam it, microwave it or bake it.

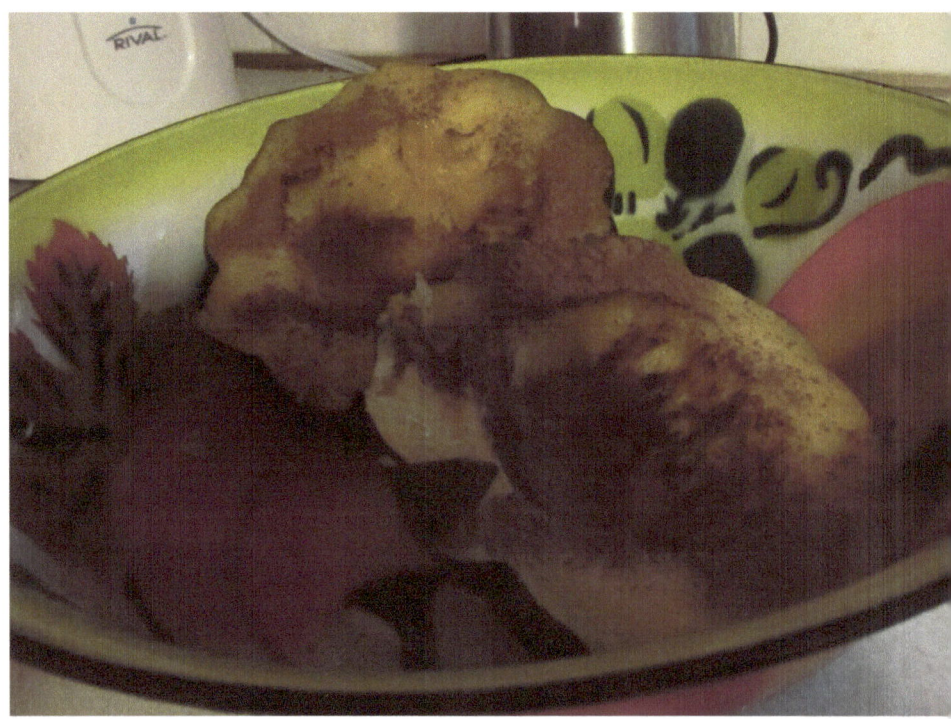

I love to steam veggies because I use the leftover water to start my next soup

Those vitamins left from the cooking are in the water, making a wonderful start for your next soup. Steaming an acorn squash depends on its size. An average squash takes about 20 minutes to steam and about 10 minutes in the microwave, so steaming (a better natural way is the best).

With steaming or microwaving, just stick a fork in to test! And always cook the squash whole and washed with a few fork pricks throughout the squash.

For toppings- after cooled, cut in half and empty the seeds, sprinkle some cinnamon and stevia if you like it sweet. But it has a natural sweetness so you probably just need some spices of your choice like cinnamon.

Lentil and Sweet Potato Burgers

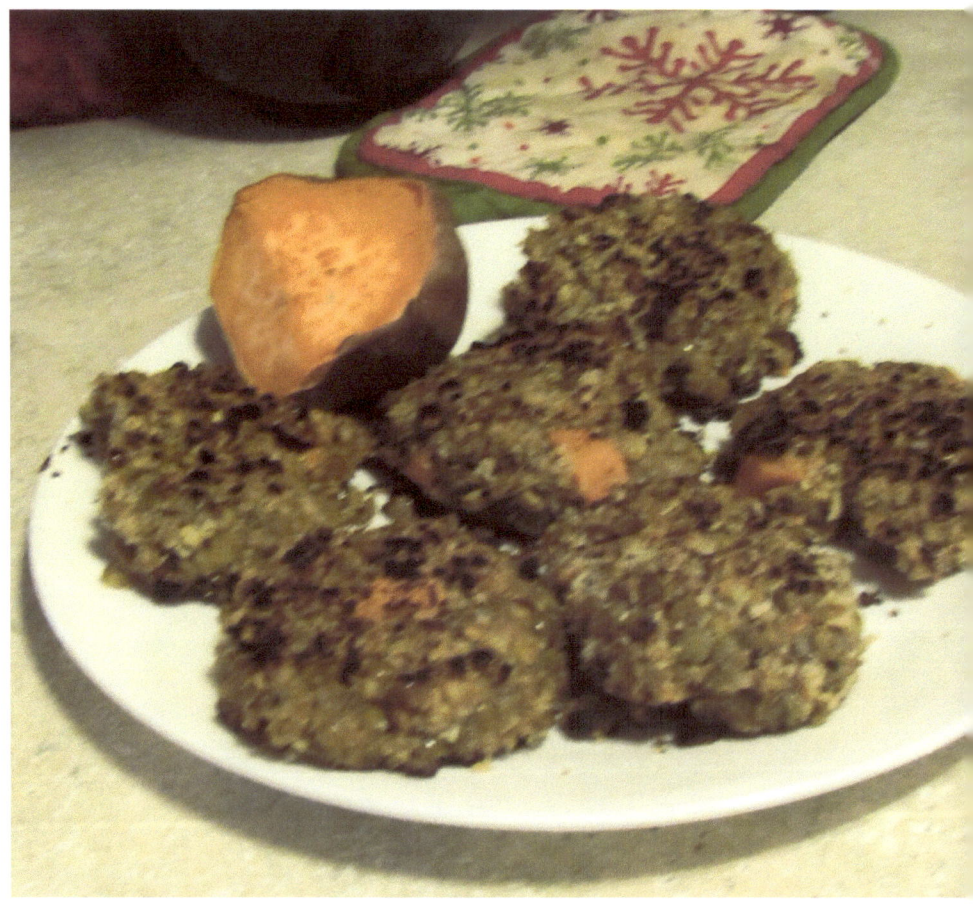

Making your own veggie burgers can be difficult because it is hard to make them stick together and then cook on a grill or frying pan

I have been trying for years to perfect the veggie burger,

especially in the summer time when I would like to have a burger with my friends who eat meat.

Cook 1 cup Lentils and allow cooling.

Lentils are a legume which is very healthy for you, packed with protein – 8 grams per serving. Cook following directions on the package but most legumes, like rice or any other grain, take 1 cup of water to 1 cup of legumes, bringing water to a boil and adding lentils, lowering to a simmer and cooking for about 10-12 minutes. I like my lentils firm, not soft. It works better if you undercook them a bit so that you can still see the circular lentil.

Next:

Finely chop a clove of fresh garlic and chunk of fresh ginger

Chop a small red onion

Cube an already partially cooked small sweet potato. You do not want the potato soft, it needs to be firm. You can also use a white potato. The starch in white potatoes helps the lentils to gather together.

In a mixing bowl, mix lentils sweet potatoes, fresh garlic and ginger, adding 1 teaspoon of soy sauce and 1/2 cup whole wheat bread crumbs. If you want the burgers smoother you can put mixture into a food processor for a different texture.

Form into patties and then use another ½ cup of bread crumbs to coat each veggie burger to help them with crispness on the outside.

Cook and flip in frying pan with 1 teaspoon of olive oil for 10 minutes.

Serve with whole grain bread and toppings such as lettuce and tomato.

The health and wellness benefits of whole grains

Did you know that sweet corn is a grain? Most people think of corn on the cob as a veggie. Even in the can, corn can be a great addition to your diet. You just have to limit portion sizes because of its sweetness.

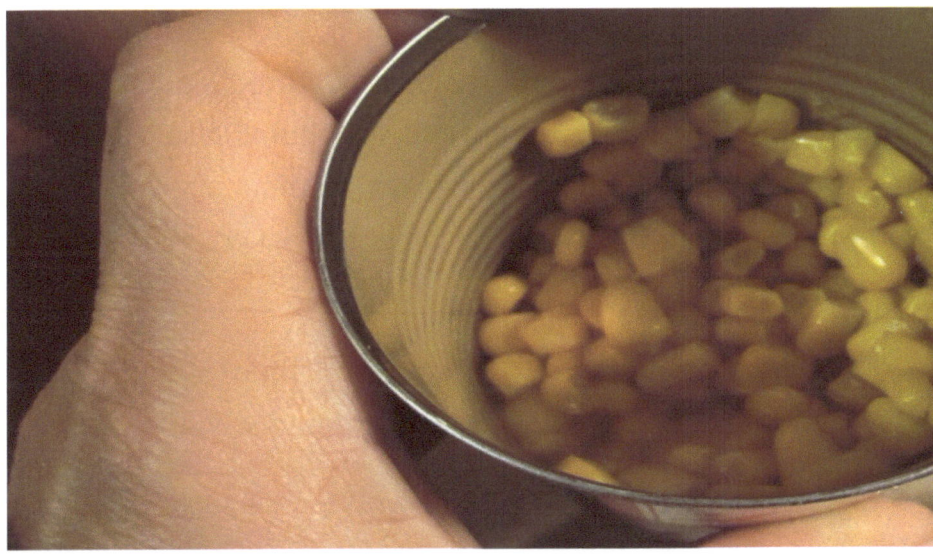

Sweet corn is immature, and enjoyed as a vegetable rather than being left to dry and used as a grain.

Popcorn is a grain with a hard hull which pops because steam builds up inside of the hull.

Polenta is a coarse meal eaten as soft mush that is dried and then fried. In Italy polenta may be made with other ingredients such as farro or chestnut flour.

Polenta cooked has a smooth creamy texture but when cooked it can be sliced into wedges or sticks and then pan fried.

List of other grains

Amaranth, barley, corn (including whole cornmeal and popcorn), millet, oats (including oatmeal), quinoa, rice; both brown and colored rice, Sorghum (also called milo) Rye, and wheat; including spelt, emmer, farro, einkorn, durum and forms such as bulgur, cracked wheat and wheat berries, and wild rice.

What people seem to be confused about is the difference between whole wheat and whole grain.

Whole wheat is one kind of whole grain, so all whole wheat is whole grain, but not all whole grain is whole wheat!

The definition of Whole Grains: Whole grains or foods made from them contain all the essential parts and naturally occurring nutrients of the entire grain seed in their original proportions. If the grain has been processed, (cracked, crushed, rolled, extruded and/or cooked), the food product should deliver the same rich balance of nutrients that are found in the original grain seed.

Definition of whole grains-taken from: The Whole GrainsCouncil:http://wholegrainscouncil.org/whole-grains-101/definition-of- whole-grains

Some Whole Grain Side Dishes- Quinoa

 You cook quinoa just as you do rice; equal portions of water to quinoa

Dessert Quinoa

I like to make dessert quinoa or as a side dish and all I have to do is cook equal parts of water to quinoa, bring to a boil and simmer. Then when it cools I add my favorite spices such as cinnamon and stevia if I want it sweet. I also add chopped apples, a ½ cup of plain coconut yogurt and top my quinoa with sliced pineapple.

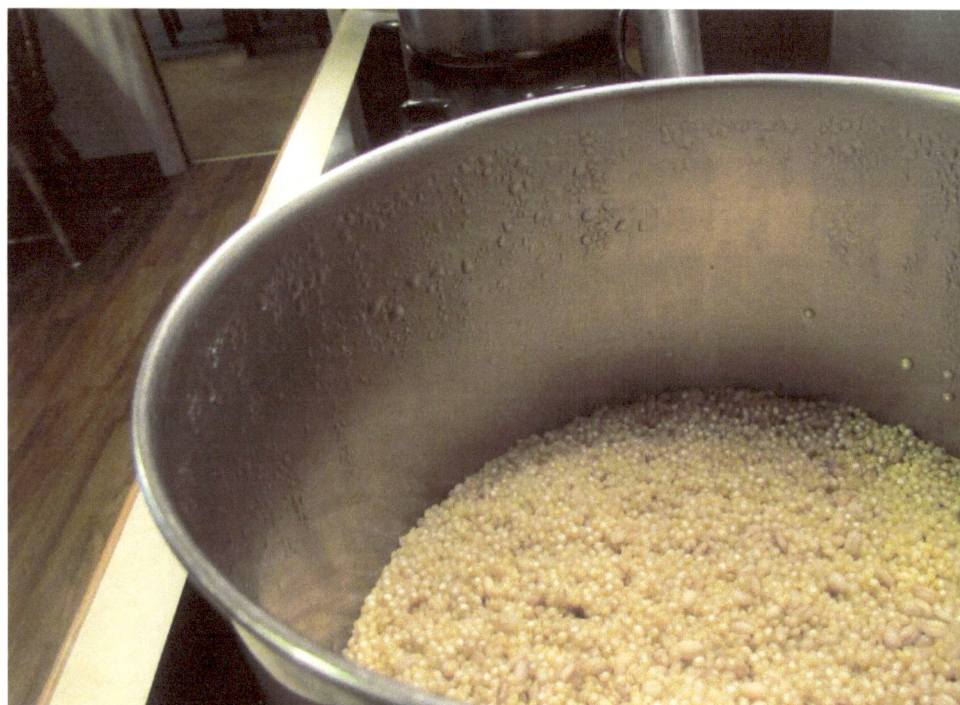

Side Dish Quinoa

If you want your quinoa to be for a side dish or meal for lunch or dinner, add chopped carrots, chopped olives, celery and onions. I also add other veggies such as spinach or broccoli. If you want more moisture to your quinoa add some vegetable broth.

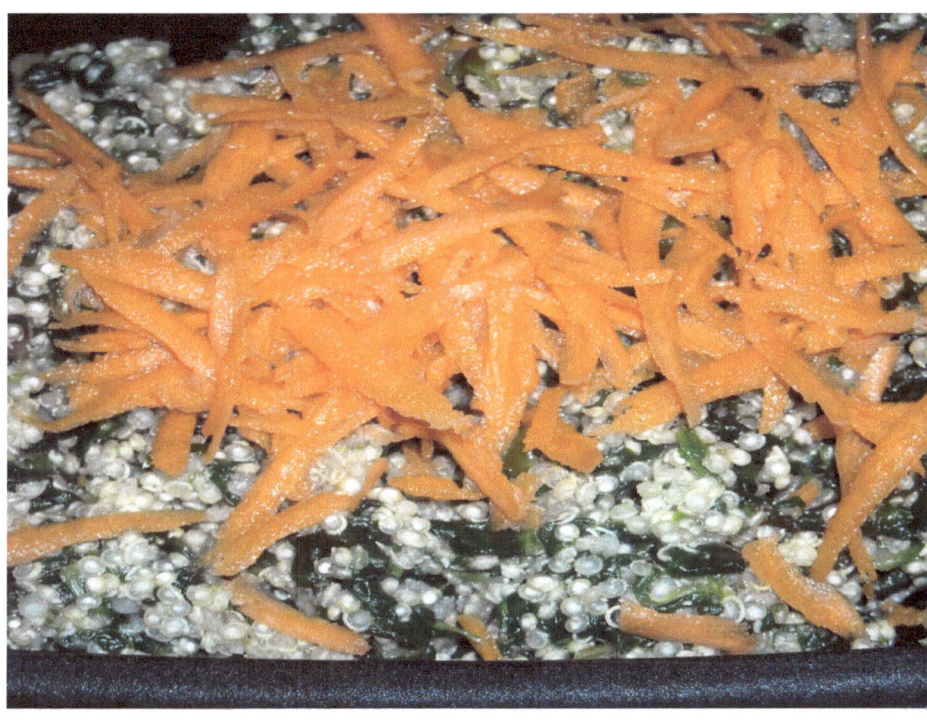

Quinoa side dish for lunch or dinner

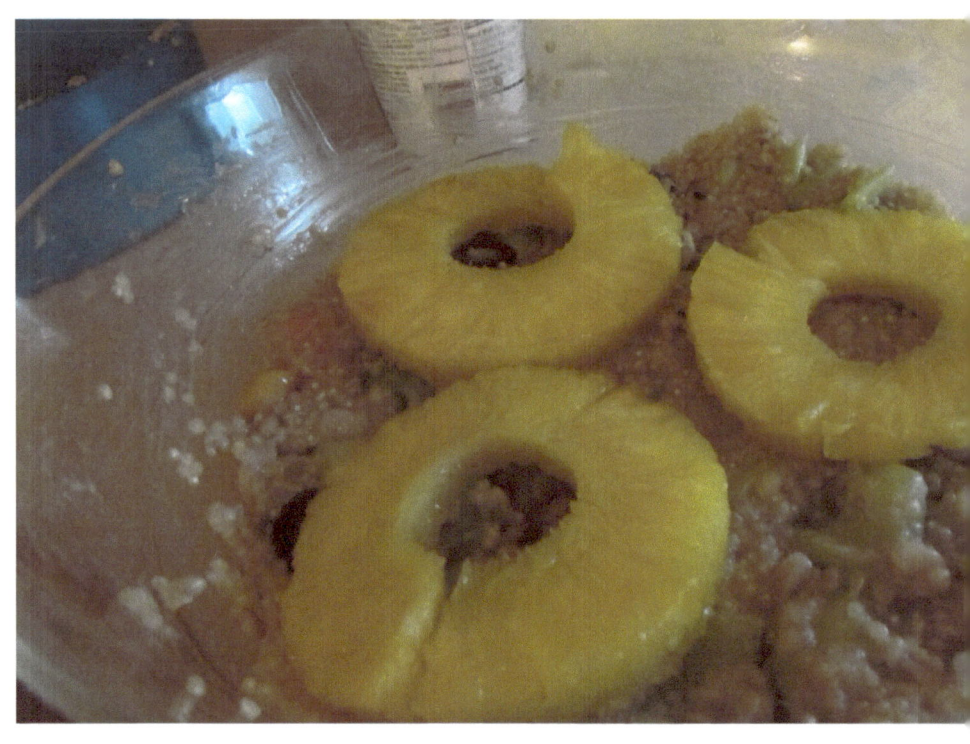

Quinoa topped with sliced pineapple

Baked or Simmered Tofu

There are basics to vegetarian and vegan cooking methods; one of them is to learn about cooking tofu.

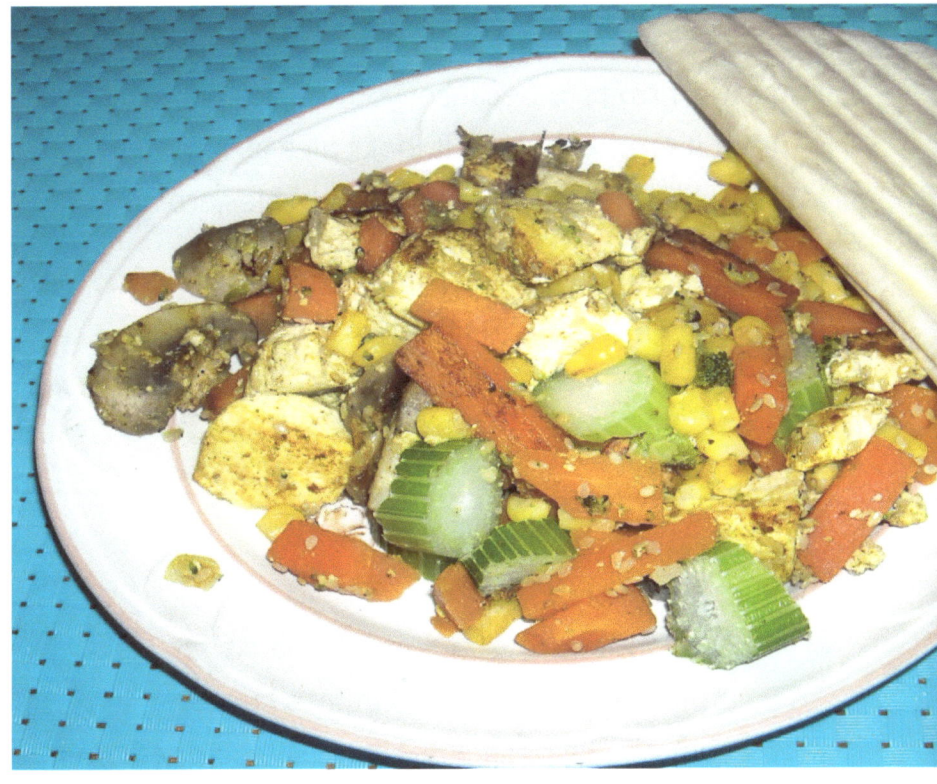

After cooking tofu in a frying pan with some olive oil (or canola oil spray) you have a great meal. This meal has fennel, mushrooms red peppers and yellow corn added to the tofu

Tofu is packed with protein, and a great replacement to eating meat, so learn how to cook it if you want some added protein in your diet that is not meat. Just like grains, tofu has about 9 grams of protein per serving. Basic ways to cook tofu: baked and simmered in a frying pan.

Use extra firm tofu because you can cube it easily without it crumbling and it looks nice as a perfect looking dish once cooked and vegetables are added.

Marinade is important to tofu because it takes on the flavor of what you marinade it in.

Marinade:

1. Cup of vegetable broth
2. 1 clove chopped garlic
3. 1 piece chopped ginger
4. 2 teaspoons low sodium soy sauce
5. 1 block extra firm tofu cut into cubes
6. Your choice of spices- I love using curry, cumin and turmeric because the tofu turns a bright yellow color

Marinade for at least 1 hour. If you marinade overnight it really soaks into the tofu.

Before I gather the vegetables that I am planning for my meal, I cook the tofu; either baking it in a 350 degree oven for about 20 minutes on a canola sprayed cookie sheet, or in a frying pan, gently stirring, browning well on each side. You can also roll your tofu into bread crumbs before cooking for a crisper taste. I then add the veggies I love such as broccoli, carrots, and spinach. Cook another 10 minutes depending on the texture that you like your veggies.

I hope that this booklet helps you move toward a healthier plant based diet. Begin to experiment as I have with different ingredients and foods. Just recently, I discovered the parsnip, and I love its flavor and texture.

Happy Cooking!

Doris

www.ingramcontent.com/pod-product-compliance
Lightning Source LLC
Chambersburg PA
CBHW051128290526
45796CB00001B/5